THE FASTEST WAY TO MOTHERHOOD

Proven Tips For Boosting Fertility And Conceiving Quickly

Judith J Ellis

DISCLAIMER

All rights reserved. Do not republish any part of this book publication in any form or by any means, including scanning, photocopying or otherwise, without prior written permission to the copyright holder.

ISBN: 9798374369564

Imprint: Independently published

Content

Introduction

Becoming a mother is one of the most fulfilling experiences a woman can have, but for some, the journey to conception can be a long and difficult one. If you're looking to boost your fertility and increase your chances of conceiving quickly, you're not alone. Fortunately, there are many proven methods for maximizing your fertility and speeding up the process of becoming pregnant. In this guide, we'll explore the most effective tips and strategies for boosting your fertility and achieving a successful pregnancy as quickly as possible. From lifestyle changes to medical interventions, we'll cover all the options available to help you on your journey to motherhood.

Chapter One

Understanding Fertility: The Basics Of Conception And Reproductive Health

This chapter will provide a general overview of the biological processes that are involved in conception and pregnancy. It will cover topics such as the menstrual cycle, ovulation, fertilization, and implantation. It will also explain the various factors that can affect fertility, including age, genetics, and underlying health conditions. Additionally, it will discuss common fertility tests and assessments that are used to evaluate a person's fertility potential.

- **The Menstrual Cycle and Ovulation:**

The menstrual cycle is the regular series of changes that happen in a woman's body in preparation for pregnancy. The menstrual cycle is controlled by hormones that regulate the growth and shedding of the uterine lining. The menstrual cycle typically lasts 28 days, but it can vary from 21 to 35 days. Ovulation is the process where a mature egg is released from the ovary and travels down the Fallopian tube, where it may be fertilized by sperm. Understanding when you ovulate is critical to understanding your fertile window.

- **Fertilization and Implantation:**

Once the egg is released from the ovary, it travels down the Fallopian tube where it may be fertilized by sperm. Fertilization takes place whilst the sperm enters the egg.. The fertilized egg then travels to the uterus and implants in the lining of the uterus, where it begins to grow and develop into a fetus.

- **Factors that affect fertility:**

There are many factors that can affect fertility, including age, genetics, and underlying health conditions. Age is a significant factor in fertility, as a woman's fertility begins to decline in her late twenties. Genetics can also play a role in fertility, as certain genetic conditions can affect the ability to conceive. Health conditions such as polycystic ovary syndrome (PCOS), endometriosis, and thyroid disorders can also affect fertility.

- **Fertility tests and assessments**:

Fertility tests and assessments are used to evaluate a person's fertility potential. These tests can include blood tests to measure hormone levels, ultrasound exams to evaluate the ovaries and uterus, and diagnostic procedures such as hysterosalpingography (HSG) and laparoscopy to evaluate the Fallopian tubes and ovaries.

- **Age and fertility:** Age is one of the most significant factors that affect fertility. As a woman gets older, her fertility naturally declines, and the chances of conceiving decrease. The peak of a woman's fertility is in her late teens and early twenties, and it gradually declines as she approaches her thirties. By the time a woman reaches her early forties, her fertility has dropped significantly, and the chances of conceiving are very low. It's important for women to be aware of their age-related fertility decline and plan accordingly.

- **Genetic factors:**

Genetics can also play a role in fertility. Certain genetic conditions can affect the ability to conceive. For example, Turner syndrome and Klinefelter syndrome are genetic conditions that affect women and men, respectively, and can lead to infertility. Genetic testing can help identify these conditions and allow couples to make informed decisions about their fertility options.

- **Health conditions and fertility:**

Certain health conditions can also affect fertility. Polycystic ovary syndrome (PCOS) is a common condition that affects women and can lead to infertility. Endometriosis, a condition where the tissue that lines the uterus grows outside of it, can also affect fertility. Thyroid disorders, such as hypothyroidism and hyperthyroidism, can also affect fertility. It's important for couples to be aware of any underlying health conditions that may affect their fertility and to seek medical help if needed.

- **Fertility tests and assessments**: Fertility tests and assessments are used to evaluate a person's fertility potential. These tests can include blood tests to measure hormone levels, ultrasound exams to evaluate the ovaries and uterus, and diagnostic procedures such as hysterosalpingography (HSG) and laparoscopy to evaluate the Fallopian tubes and ovaries. These tests can help identify any potential issues that may be affecting fertility, and allow couples to make informed decisions about their fertility options.

You will gain a thorough understanding of the fundamentals of fertility and the variables that can influence it after reading this chapter. You will also have a better understanding of the many fertility tests and evaluations that are available and how to utilize them to estimate a person's fertility potential. As you continue on your path to parenthood and choose your reproductive options, having this knowledge will be essential to you.

Chapter Two

Lifestyle Changes For Boosting Fertility: Diet, Exercise, And Stress Management

The emphasis of this chapter will be on modifying one's lifestyle to increase fertility. It will go over issues including how crucial it is to keep a good diet, engage in regular exercise, and control your stress. It will also go through how these lifestyle modifications might assist boost fertility and raise the likelihood of conceiving rapidly.

- **The Importance Of A Healthy Diet:**

  Eating a healthy diet that is rich in nutrients can help boost fertility. This includes consuming plenty of fruits and vegetables, lean protein, and healthy fats. It's also important to avoid processed foods and excessive alcohol consumption. Eating a balanced diet can help regulate hormones and maintain a healthy weight, which can improve fertility.

- **The Benefits Of Regular Exercise:**

Regular exercise can also help boost fertility. Exercise can help regulate hormones, maintain a healthy weight, and improve overall physical and mental well-being. However, it's important to avoid over-exercising, which can have the opposite effect on fertility.

- **Managing Stress Levels:**

Stress can affect fertility. Chronic stress can affect hormones and impede ovulation. It's important to find ways to manage stress, such as through meditation, yoga, or therapy.

- **How Lifestyle Changes Can Improve Fertility:**

Making lifestyle changes, such as eating a healthy diet, getting regular exercise, and managing stress levels can have a positive impact on fertility. These changes can help regulate hormones, maintain a healthy weight, and improve overall physical and mental well-being, which can increase the chances of conceiving quickly.

- **The Role Of Weight In Fertility:**

Weight can also have an impact on fertility. Being overweight or underweight can affect hormone levels and impede ovulation. Maintaining a healthy weight through a balanced diet and regular exercise can help regulate hormones and improve fertility.

- **The Impact Of Smoking And Alcohol Consumption On Fertility:**

Smoking and excessive alcohol consumption can negatively impact fertility. Smoking can affect the quality of eggs and sperm and decrease the chances of conception. Excessive alcohol consumption can also affect hormone levels and impede ovulation. Quitting smoking and limiting alcohol consumption can help improve fertility.

- **The Role Of Sleep In Fertility:**

: Getting adequate sleep is also important for fertility. Sleep plays a crucial role in regulating hormones, and poor sleep can affect ovulation and conception. It's important to aim for 7-8 hours of quality sleep per night and to establish a consistent sleep schedule.

- **The Importance Of Self-Care:** Self-care is also important for boosting fertility. Taking care of oneself both physically and mentally can help improve overall well-being, which can, in turn, improve fertility. Self-care can include activities such as yoga, meditation, and spending time in nature.

This chapter will provide you a thorough explanation of how lifestyle choices affect fertility as well as suggestions for adjustments that can be made. It will assist you in realizing the value of preserving a healthy weight and diet, engaging in regular exercise, controlling stress, giving up smoking and drinking only in moderation, getting enough sleep, and practicing self-care. Additionally, it will direct you in making the required changes to increase your fertility by assisting you in identifying any aspects of your lifestyle that might need improvement.

Chapter Three

Nutrition And Supplements: How They Can Boost Fertility

This chapter will focus on how nutrition and supplements can boost fertility. It will cover topics such as the importance of certain vitamins and minerals for fertility, the benefits of certain foods for fertility, and the potential risks and benefits of taking fertility supplements.

The Importance Of Certain Vitamins And Minerals For Fertility:

Certain vitamins and minerals play an important role in fertility. For example, folic acid, which is a

Type of B vitamin, is essential for the healthy development of the fetus. Iron is also important for fertility as it helps in the production of healthy red blood cells. Additionally, zinc, selenium, and vitamin E are essential for maintaining healthy sperm, and vitamin D is important for the regulation of hormones.

- **The Benefits Of Certain Foods For Fertility:**

Certain foods can also boost fertility. For example, fatty fish such as salmon and tuna are rich in omega-3 fatty acids, which are important for the health of eggs and sperm. Whole grains, fruits, and vegetables are also important for fertility, as they provide essential vitamins and minerals. Legumes, nuts, and seeds are also important for fertility as they provide healthy fats, protein, and zinc.

- **The Potential Risks And Benefits Of Taking Fertility Supplements:**

Fertility supplements are available to help boost fertility, but it's important to be aware of the potential risks and benefits. Some supplements, such as folic acid and iron, are considered safe for use during pregnancy. However, it is important to consult with a doctor before taking any fertility supplement, as some supplements may contain substances that can be harmful.

- **Addressing Specific Nutritional Deficiencies:**

It's important to identify and address any specific nutritional deficiencies that may be affecting fertility. For example, an iron deficiency can lead to anemia, which can affect ovulation. Similarly, a deficiency in vitamin D can lead to hormonal imbalances. Identifying and addressing these deficiencies through diet, supplements, or other means can help improve fertility.

- **The Role Of Antioxidant-Rich Foods In Fertility:**

Antioxidant-rich foods can also play a role in boosting fertility. Antioxidants help to protect cells from damage caused by free radicals, which can negatively impact fertility. Foods that are high in antioxidants include berries, leafy greens, nuts, and seeds.

- **The Impact Of Caffeine And Sugar On Fertility:**

Caffeine and sugar can also affect fertility. Caffeine can affect ovulation, and excessive consumption may lead to hormonal imbalances. Similarly, a high intake of sugar can lead to weight gain and affect hormone levels, which can negatively impact fertility. It's important to limit caffeine and sugar intake to improve fertility.

- **The Role Of Probiotics And Fermented Foods In Fertility:**

Probiotics and fermented foods can also play a role in boosting fertility. Probiotics are beneficial bacteria that can help to balance the gut microbiome. Fermented foods such as yogurt, kefir, and sauerkraut are also good sources of probiotics. A healthy gut microbiome is important for overall health, including reproductive health.

- **The Benefits Of A Plant-Based Diet:**

A plant-based diet has been associated with many health benefits, including improved fertility. Plant-based diets are typically high in antioxidants, fiber, and phytochemical, which can all help to improve fertility. Plant-based diets can also help to maintain a healthy weight and regulate hormones, which can improve fertility.

You will gain a thorough understanding of how nutrition and supplements might increase fertility in this chapter. You will have a better understanding of the value of particular vitamins and minerals, the advantages of particular diets, and the potential drawbacks and advantages of using fertility supplements. Additionally, it will direct you on how to adjust your diet appropriately, take supplements, or take care of any nutritional deficiencies that might be influencing your fertility. You will learn more about the effects of plant-based diets, probiotics, sugar, fermented foods, and caffeine on fertility.

Chapter Four

Fertility-Tracking And Ovulation Prediction Methods

This chapter will focus on the various methods available for tracking fertility and predicting ovulation. It will cover topics such as basal body temperature (BBT) charting, ovulation predictor kits (OPKs), and fertility apps. Additionally, it will discuss the pros and cons of each method and how they can be used effectively to increase the chances of conceiving quickly.

Basal Body Temperature (BBT) Charting:

Basal body temperature charting is a method of tracking fertility by recording the body's temperature every morning before getting out of bed. A small increase in temperature, usually around 0.2-0.5 degrees Fahrenheit, typically occurs at the time of ovulation. By charting BBT, a woman can identify her ovulation pattern and predict her fertile window.

Ovulation Predictor Kits (OPKs):

Ovulation predictor kits (OPKs) are another method of tracking fertility. These kits detect the presence of the luteinizing hormone (LH) in urine, which rises just before ovulation. By identifying this LH surge, a woman can predict when she is most likely to ovulate.

Fertility Apps:

Fertility apps are another method of tracking fertility. These apps use a combination of methods such as BBT charting, tracking of the menstrual cycle, and inputting data from ovulation predictor kits, to predict ovulation and identify fertile windows. They also provide educational resources and support, as well as the ability to track symptoms and progress over time. However, it is important to note that the accuracy of these apps may vary and it's important to consult with a healthcare professional before making any decisions based on the predictions made by these apps.

Pros and cons of fertility tracking methods:

Each method of fertility tracking has its pros and cons. BBT charting is a natural method, but it requires daily tracking and may not be as accurate as other methods. Ovulation predictor kits are easy to use and can be more accurate than BBT charting, but they can be expensive if used regularly. Fertility apps can be convenient and provide a comprehensive view of fertility data but the accuracy may vary.

Combining Fertility Tracking Methods:

Combining multiple methods of fertility tracking can be more effective than relying on one method alone. For example, by combining BBT charting with ovulation predictor kits, a woman can get a more accurate picture of her fertile window.

and how they can be used in conjunction with other methods to track fertility.

Importance Of Consulting A Healthcare Professional:

It's important to consult a healthcare professional before starting any fertility tracking method. A healthcare professional can provide guidance on which method or methods may be best suited for an individual and can also provide support and advice throughout the process.

Interpreting The Results:

Understanding how to interpret the results of fertility tracking methods is essential. A healthcare professional can help interpret the results and provide guidance on how to use them to increase the chances of conception. Additionally, it's important to note that fertility tracking methods should be used as a guide and that other factors, such as age, underlying health conditions, and the duration of time trying to conceive, should also be taken into consideration when interpreting results.

When To Seek Medical Help:

If a woman has been tracking her fertility for several months without success, it may be time to seek medical help. A healthcare professional can perform further testing to determine if there are any underlying fertility issues and can provide advice on fertility treatments if needed.

You will gain a thorough understanding of the numerous techniques for monitoring fertility and forecasting ovulation from this chapter. You will learn about the benefits and drawbacks of each technique, how to utilize them to improve your chances of getting pregnant quickly, the significance of consulting a healthcare professional, how to interpret the results, and when to seek medical attention. Additionally, it will assist you in making knowledgeable decisions about your fertility and raise your chances of conceiving a child.

Chapter Five

Maximizing Your Chances Of Conceiving: Timing, Ovulation, And Intercourse

This chapter will focus on the importance of timing, ovulation, and intercourse in increasing the chances of conception. It will cover topics such as the fertile window, the best positions for intercourse, and the role of sperm in conception. Additionally, it will discuss the importance of having regular intercourse throughout the menstrual cycle to increase the chances of conception.

The Fertile Window:

The fertile window is the period when a woman is most likely to conceive. It typically occurs around the time of ovulation, when an egg is released from the ovary. By identifying the fertile window, a couple can increase their chances of conception by having intercourse during this time.

The Best Positions For Intercourse:

Certain positions for intercourse can also increase the chances of conception. Positions that allow for deep penetration, such as the missionary position, can help to deposit sperm closer to the cervix, increasing the chances of fertilization. Additionally, positions that allow for the retention of semen, such as the spooning position, can also increase the chances of conception.

The Role Of Sperm In Conception:

Sperm play an important role in conception. They must be able to reach and fertilize the egg for conception to occur. Factors such as sperm count, motility, and morphology can affect the chances of conception. It's important to address any issues with sperm quality with a healthcare professional.

The Importance Of Regular Intercourse Throughout The Menstrual Cycle:

Having regular intercourse throughout the menstrual cycle can also increase the chances of conception. This helps to ensure that sperm are present when the egg is released, increasing the chances of fertilization. Additionally, having regular intercourse can also help to identify the fertile window and increase the chances of conception.

Understanding Ovulation And Its Timing:

Ovulation is the process of the release of an egg from the ovary. Understanding the timing of ovulation is important for increasing the chances of conception. Ovulation typically occurs around 14 days before the start of the next menstrual cycle, but this can vary from woman to woman. Understanding the timing of ovulation can be done by tracking basal body temperature, using ovulation predictor kits, or monitoring cervical mucus, among other methods.

Importance Of Cervical Mucus:

Cervical mucus plays an important role in fertility. The cervical mucus changes throughout the menstrual cycle, becoming more fertile and more favorable for sperm survival as ovulation approaches. By monitoring cervical mucus, a woman can identify her fertile window and increase her chances of conception.

Intercourse Frequency And Timing:

The frequency and timing of intercourse can also affect the chances of conception. It's recommended to have intercourse every other day leading up to ovulation, as sperm can survive for up to five days in the female reproductive tract. This helps to ensure that sperm are present when the egg is released, increasing the chances of fertilization.

Addressing Any Fertility-Related Issues:

If a couple has been trying to conceive for several months without success, it may be necessary to address any fertility-related issues. A healthcare professional can perform further testing to determine if there are any underlying fertility issues and can provide advice on fertility treatments if needed.

This chapter will provide you with a comprehensive understanding of the importance of timing, ovulation, and intercourse in increasing the chances of conception. It will help you understand the fertile window, the best positions for intercourse, the role of sperm in conception, the importance of cervical mucus, and the intercourse frequency and timing. It will also guide you to make informed decisions about your fertility, address any fertility-related issues, and increase your chances of successful conception.

Chapter Six

Navigating The Journey To Motherhood: Coping With Infertility And Making Informed Decisions

This chapter will focus on the emotional and psychological aspects of navigating the journey to motherhood, specifically coping with infertility and making informed decisions about fertility treatments. It will cover topics such as the emotional impact of infertility, the different types of fertility treatments available, and the importance of making informed decisions about treatments.

The Emotional Impact Of Infertility:

Infertility can have a significant emotional impact on individuals and couples. It can lead to feelings of sadness, frustration, guilt, and even depression. It's important to address the emotional aspects of infertility and to seek support from a healthcare professional or counselor.

The Different Types Of Fertility Treatments Available:

There are various types of fertility treatments available, including medications, surgery, artificial insemination, and assisted reproductive technologies (ART) such as in-vitro fertilization (IVF). It's important to understand the different options available and to consult with a healthcare professional to determine the best course of treatment.

The Importance Of Making Informed Decisions About Treatments:

It's important to make informed decisions about fertility treatments. This includes understanding the risks, benefits, and success rates of each treatment, as well as the potential emotional and financial impact. Consultation with a healthcare professional and/or a fertility specialist can help in making informed decisions.

Coping With The Emotional Aspects Of Fertility Treatments:

Fertility treatments can also have an emotional impact. The process of undergoing treatments can be stressful and can lead to feelings of disappointment and discouragement if the treatments are not successful. It's important to have a support system in place and to seek help from a healthcare professional or counselor if needed.

Considering Alternatives:

If fertility treatments are not successful, it's important to consider alternatives such as adoption or surrogacy. It's also important to understand that parenting can take many forms and that there are many paths to building a family.

The Role Of Support Groups And Community Resources:

Support groups and community resources can also help navigate the journey to motherhood. Support groups provide a platform for individuals and couples to connect with others who are also facing similar struggles with infertility. They can provide emotional support and can also serve as a source of information about fertility treatments and other options for building a family. Community resources such as clinics and support organizations can also provide information and support for individuals and couples dealing with infertility.

The Importance Of Open Communication With Your Partner:

Open communication with your partner is crucial when navigating the journey to motherhood. Infertility can place a strain on relationships, and it's important to discuss feelings and concerns with your partner. This can help to maintain intimacy and strengthen the relationship.

The Decision To Stop Treatment:

It's important to consider the decision to stop fertility treatments. This decision can be difficult, but it's important to consider the emotional, physical, and financial aspects. It's also important to understand that it's okay to stop treatment and explore other options for building a family.

This chapter will provide you with a comprehensive understanding of the emotional and psychological aspects of navigating the journey to motherhood, specifically coping with infertility and making informed decisions about fertility treatments. It will help you understand the emotional impact of infertility, the different types of fertility treatments available, the importance of making informed decisions about treatments, coping with the emotional aspects of fertility treatments, considering alternatives, the role of support groups and community resources, the importance of open communication with your partner and the decision to stop treatment. It will also guide you to make informed decisions about your fertility, address any emotional and psychological issues, and find the path that works

best for you in building a family.

Chapter Seven

Fertility Treatments: Understanding The Pros And Cons

This chapter will focus on the various fertility treatments available and the pros and cons of each. It will cover topics such as medications, surgery, artificial insemination, and assisted reproductive technologies (ART) such as in-vitro fertilization (IVF). Additionally, it will discuss the potential risks and benefits of each treatment and the success rates associated with each.

Medications:

Fertility medications, such as clomiphene citrate (Clomid) and gonadotropins, are commonly used to stimulate ovulation. These medications can be effective in increasing the chances of conception, but they can also come with potential side effects such as hot flashes and mood swings. Additionally, these medications may not be suitable for women with certain underlying health conditions.

Surgery:

Fertility surgery is another option for treating infertility. Surgery can be used to correct structural problems such as blockages in the fallopian tubes or to remove endometriosis. Surgery can be effective in increasing the chances of conception, but it can also come with risks such as infection and bleeding.

Artificial Insemination:

Artificial insemination is a procedure in which sperm is inserted into the uterus using a small catheter. This procedure can be effective in increasing the chances of conception, but it may not be suitable for couples with certain underlying fertility issues.

Assisted Reproductive Technologies (ART):

Assisted reproductive technologies (ART) such as in-vitro fertilization (IVF) involve the fertilization of an egg outside of the body, followed by the transfer of the embryo to the uterus. IVF and other ART techniques can be effective in increasing the chances of conception, but they can also come with risks such as multiple pregnancies and ovarian hyperstimulation syndrome (OHSS).

The Importance Of Considering All Options:

It's important to consider all fertility treatment options and to consult with a healthcare professional to determine the best course of treatment. Each treatment has its pros and cons, and it's important to weigh these against the chances of success before making a decision.

The Cost And Accessibility Of Fertility Treatments:

Cost and accessibility are also important factors to consider when it comes to fertility treatments. Some treatments, such as medications and artificial insemination, may be more affordable than others, such as IVF. Insurance coverage for fertility treatments can vary greatly and it's important to understand the coverage and costs associated with each treatment. Additionally, some treatments may not be readily available in certain areas, and it's important to consider the accessibility of different treatments.

The Emotional and Psychological Impact Of Fertility Treatments:

Fertility treatments can also have an emotional and psychological impact. The process of undergoing treatments can be stressful, and the pressure to conceive can take a toll on individuals and couples. It's important to have a support system in place and to seek help from a healthcare professional or counselor if needed.

The Decision To Stop Treatment:

Ultimately, it's important to consider the decision to stop fertility treatments. This decision can be difficult, but it's important to consider the emotional, physical, financial, and accessibility aspects. It's also important to understand that it's okay to stop treatment and explore other options for building a family.

This chapter will provide y with you a comprehensive understanding of the various fertility treatments available and the pros and cons of each. It will help you understand the potential risks and benefits, success rates, cost, and accessibility of each treatment. It will also guide you to make informed decisions about your fertility treatments, by considering all options, the risks and benefits, consulting with a healthcare professional, understanding the emotional and psychological impact of fertility treatments, and the decision to stop treatment. It will also help you explore other options for building a family.

Chapter eight

Support And Resources: Finding Help And Information On Your Path To Conception

We shall be focusing on the importance of support and resources in navigating the journey to motherhood. It will cover topics such as support groups, community resources, and online resources for finding information and help. Additionally, it will discuss the importance of having a support system in place and seeking help when needed.

Support Groups:

Support groups can provide a platform for individuals and couples to connect with others who are also facing similar struggles with infertility. They can provide emotional support and can also serve as a source of information about fertility treatments and other options for building a family.

Community Resources:

Community resources such as clinics and support organizations can also provide information and support for individuals and couples dealing with infertility. They can also provide information on local support groups and other resources.

Online Resources:

There are also numerous online resources available for finding information and help on the journey to motherhood. Websites and forums can provide information on fertility treatments, as well as emotional support and advice from others who have gone through similar experiences.

The Importance Of Having A Support System In Place:

Having a support system in place is essential when navigating the journey to motherhood. This can include friends, family, a partner, a healthcare professional, or a counselor. They can provide emotional support and help to navigate the process of fertility treatments and other options for building a family.

Seeking Help When Needed:

It's important to seek help when needed. This can include consulting with a healthcare professional, seeking counseling or therapy, or joining a support group. It's important to address any emotional or psychological issues that may arise during the journey to motherhood.

Consulting With A Fertility Specialist:

Consulting with a fertility specialist can also provide valuable information and support for individuals and couples dealing with infertility. Fertility specialists can provide personalized advice and treatment options, as well as help navigate the process of fertility treatments.

Financial And Legal Resources:

Financial and legal resources are also important to consider when navigating the journey to motherhood. This can include information on insurance coverage for fertility treatments, as well as resources for financial assistance and legal support for adoption or surrogacy.

Self-Care And Self-Compassion:

Self-care and self-compassion are crucial when navigating the journey to motherhood. It's important to take care of oneself emotionally and physically and to practice self-compassion. This can include engaging in self-care activities such as exercise, yoga, or meditation.

This chapter will provide you with a comprehensive understanding of the importance of support and resources in navigating the journey to motherhood. It will help you understand the various resources available such as support groups, community resources, online resources, consulting with a fertility specialist, financial and legal resources, and the importance of self-care and self-compassion. It will also guide you to make informed decisions about your fertility, address any emotional and psychological issues, and find the path that works best for you in building a family. It will also emphasize the importance of having a support system in place and seeking help when needed.

Chapter Nine

Conclusion: Putting It All Together And Moving Forward On Your Journey To Motherhood

This chapter will serve as a conclusion to the book, bringing together all of the information and advice presented in the previous chapters. It will summarize the key takeaways and provide readers with a plan for moving forward on their journey to motherhood.

Understanding Fertility:

The first step in increasing the chances of conception is understanding fertility. This includes understanding the basics of conception and reproductive health, as well as tracking ovulation and identifying the fertile window.

Lifestyle Changes:

Making lifestyle changes such as eating a balanced diet, exercising regularly, and managing stress can also help to boost fertility. Additionally, taking the right nutrition and supplements can also enhance fertility.

Fertility Treatments:

Fertility treatments can also be an effective way to increase the chances of conception. However, it's important to understand the pros and cons of each treatment and to make informed decisions about which treatments to pursue.

Support And Resources:

Having a support system in place and seeking help when needed is crucial when navigating the journey to motherhood. There are numerous support groups, community resources, and online resources available to provide information and support.

Emotional And Psychological Well-Being:

The journey to motherhood can be emotional and stressful. It is important to take care of oneself emotionally and physically and to practice self-compassion. This can include engaging in self-care activities such as exercise, yoga, or meditation.

Moving Forward:

Ultimately, it's important to remember that there are many paths to motherhood and to explore all options available. This may include fertility treatments, adoption, or surrogacy.

Creating A Personalized Plan:

It's important to create a personalized plan that takes into account the individual's fertility status, lifestyle, emotional and financial factors, and personal preferences. This plan should include steps to increase the chances of conception, such as making lifestyle changes and tracking ovulation, as well as a plan for pursuing fertility treatments if necessary.

Be Open To Change:

It's important to be open to change and to be flexible in one's approach. The journey to motherhood can be unpredictable and there may be unexpected turns. It's important to be prepared for the possibility that the original plan may not work out and to be open to other options such as adoption or surrogacy.

Remember To Take Care Of Yourself:

It's important to remember to take care of yourself during this journey. Whether it's seeking support from a counselor, taking time for self-care, or finding ways to manage stress, making time for yourself is essential for maintaining emotional and physical well-being.

Keep An Open Mind:

It's important to keep an open mind and to be patient. It can take time to conceive and it's important to remember that every person's journey is unique. Keep in mind that there are many paths to motherhood, and it's important to explore all options available.

This chapter will provide you with a comprehensive understanding of the journey to motherhood and a plan for moving forward. It will summarize the key takeaways from the previous chapters, guide you to make informed decisions about your fertility, address any emotional and psychological issues, and create a personalized plan. It will also emphasize the importance of being open to change, remembering to take care of yourself, keeping an open mind, and being patient. It will also guide you to explore all options available for building a family.